Weight Lifting

Basic Moves for Effective Training for Muscle Building in the Minimum Time!

Dennis E. Bradford, Ph.D.

Publisher's Notes

Conesus Lake, New York

Related Books by the Same Author

THE BEST WAY TO LOSE BODY FAT AND KEEP IT OFF!

THE 5 SECRETS TO MAKING FAST CHANGES FOR GOOD!

EMOTIONAL EMPOWERMENT

HOW TO DISSOLVE UNWANTED EMOTIONS

PERSONAL TRANSFORMATION

COMPULSIVE OVEREATING HELP

GETTING THINGS DONE

EMOTIONAL EATING

MASTERY IN 7 STEPS

Table of Contents

1: Introduction

Weight lifting is a wonderful habit. Really, it's a wonderful hobby. Since there's always something new to understand and test, it engages the mind as well as the body. It's physical and psychological benefits are so valuable that, if you are able to do it and are not doing it, you are cheating yourself.

It doesn't matter whether you are 16 or 96, male or female, young or old, fat or thin, or anywhere in between.

There are many different motivations for weightlifting. I approach it in this book from a particular angle that I suggest that you, too, adopt. *Weightlifting is important for aging physically as well as possible.*

We are all aging. Do you want to age well or poorly? Unless we decide on suicide, we don't have a choice about whether or not we want to age, but we do have plenty of choices about whether we are willing to do what it takes to age well rather than poorly.

With respect to aging physically, there are four critical habits: eating well, exercising well, supplementing well, and getting at least yearly check-ups from a medical professional that include a check of your hormone levels. Weight lifting is one kind of exercise. I discuss other kinds of exercise as well as the other habits elsewhere both online and in other books [see the Selected Bibliography].

It's impossible to age well physically unless you avoid the common epidemics of cardiovascular disease, type II diabetes, cancer, hypertension, and obesity. Although you have almost certainly heard a lot about them, you are probably less familiar with another common epidemic called "sarcopenia." Like the others, at least until the very end, it is preventable.

Sarcopenia is the loss of muscle tissue and muscular function (particularly strength) due to aging. Engaging regularly in proper weightlifting (resistance training, strength training, bodybuilding) is the best way to prevent sarcopenia. Why?

Here's a helpful analogy. Osteoporosis is having brittle, fragile bony tissue due to loss of bone mass from aging. This is an important reason why, if you are under 40, you should eat and exercise well in order to establish a reserve of bony tissue to retard or prevent osteoporosis as you age. It's an important reason why, if you are over 40, you should eat and exercise well in order to preserve as much bony tissue as possible for as long as possible. (Many people think of bones as nonliving tissues, but they are not.)

It works the same way with muscle tissue. If you are under 40, it's important to eat and exercise well in order to establish a reserve of muscle tissue to retard or prevent sarcopenia as you age. It's an important reason why, if you are over 40, you should eat and exercise well in order to preserve as much muscle tissue as possible for as long as possible.

Exercising well includes weight lifting. So, as long as you are physically able and an adult, which means here 16 years old or older, you should be eating and exercising well—including doing weightlifting--if you want to age physically as well as possible. (Actually, if you are 15 or younger, you should also eat and exercise well, too, but weight lifting using free weights or resistance machines is best avoided because your bones are not yet sufficiently developed. So wait until you are 16 to do weight lifting using free weights or resistance machines, though there's nothing wrong with getting started with bodyweight exercises such as chin-ups and push-ups and, if you are athletic, playing sports that require physical activity.)

The future is unknown and unknowable. It follows that it's impossible to know the future consequences of our present actions or inactions.

So the best way to take the best possible care of the future is to live as well as possible in the present moment. This task is to live as fully *in* the present moment as possible without merely living *for* the present moment.

If you are normal, it's likely that you could do better with respect to weightlifting, which is probably why you purchased this book.

Permit me to encourage you with some really **good news: you can obtain all the benefits from weightlifting that are necessary for aging well physically in just one or two 10-minute workouts weekly!** Of course, if you want to do more training for additional benefits, that's fine. However, if you are able-bodied and telling yourself that you are unable to lift weights for 10 or 20 minutes weekly, you are lying to yourself. Why not treat yourself more kindly?

Whether it's fitness training or weightlifting, physical exercise is most beneficial when it is intense. That's why both fitness training and weight lifting workouts should be brief. Intensity and duration are inversely proportional.

Weight lifting is a privilege. It's not a right. There are plenty of crippled people who would love to be able to do it. If you need some initial motivation, just imagine yourself being physically unable to lift weights and be grateful for the opportunity.

I assume in this book that either you have never done any weight lifting or that you haven't done it in a long time. Either way, just realize that it'll take a few months for you to get into the full swing of it.

If you are already an intermediate or advanced trainee, good for you! Although this is not a book designed for you, my hope and belief is that you'll nevertheless find some helpful tips in it.

It's important to begin by obtaining the blessing, based on a thorough physical examination, of your licensed physician in advance. The reason is that you are unique. There may be weight lifting exercises that, while beneficial to most people, would be counter-productive in your case.

Entering a noisy gym can be both intimidating and confusing. Assuming that you get the go-ahead from your physician or other licensed healthcare professional, it's important to understand exactly what to do and how to do it before lifting weights. You'll be able to begin in the privacy of your own home using as weight only your own body. Furthermore, by the time you ever enter a commercial gym, if you ever do, because you'll have read and understood this book your understanding of what to do will be better than that of many, perhaps most, trainees in the gym. So you are doing right now exactly what you should be doing.

Keep in mind that we are all different. If you and a training partner follow exactly the same routine using exactly the same poundages, your results may differ because you differ genetically. Some people gain strength and muscle faster than others. Don't worry about others. You will get stronger and more muscular if you follow the suggestions provided in this book.

Understand that it's very difficult to gain muscle. That's particularly true if you are female. There's no justification, therefore, for worrying about becoming too muscular if you are a woman. You'll only become stronger and shapelier (unless you use anabolic steroids, which are like artificial testosterone, and that's counter-productive in terms of aging well). Furthermore, muscle is several dozen times metabolically more active than fat. Therefore, you'll be able to enjoy eating more food than otherwise and, at least if you switch from burning sugar to burning fat [as I explain how to do elsewhere], your percentage of body fat will decrease naturally.

Since muscle is denser than fat, your weight may go up or stay the same as your muscle mass increases, but your percentage of body fat will decrease and you'll look better. Forget about frequently measuring your body weight; instead, once a week measure your percentage of body fat. You are too fat if it's over 20% if you are female or over 15% if you are male.

Done properly weightlifting is safe. You are not only going to be able to enjoy being stronger, looking better, and losing body fat, but you are going to obtain those goals safely if you follow the suggestions in this book.

It's important to select the right exercises and to perform them with perfect exercise technique. The right exercises are ones that are not dangerous for most people even during the long term. Many common exercises are actually dangerous. The exercises that I recommend are not dangerous for most people when performed correctly, and I explain exactly how to perform them correctly in this book. So, you will be able to lift weights safely.

As I write this, my training partner and I are relatively old. He's 68 and I'm 77. We've been training intensely nearly every week for about the last 30 years. Neither of us has ever sustained anything remotely like a serious training injury. More importantly, there's nothing unusual about that record. Unlike many of our peers, we're both relatively healthy and strong.

Do people get hurt weight lifting? Yes. However, here's an analogy that may help if you are initially concerned about safety.

Have you ever heard a landlord complain about tenant difficulties and other problems with being a landlord? I have occasionally heard such complaints. Whenever I do, I immediately understand that I'm talking to someone who is incompetent either as a real estate investor or property manager. If I'm in a certain mood, I'll ask a simple question, "How many books about it did you read before you started?" The answer, which always astounds me but shouldn't, is always "None." Mistakes in real estate can cost you tens of thousands of dollars. Personal experience is not the best teacher. Of course it takes skill to be a good landlord, but you can develop the appropriate skill set simply by reading a couple of books. Why not read before you leap?

I'm teaching to the converted. You already understand that. You're already reading a book about weightlifting before doing any. Actually, it's better to be a beginner than to be someone who started incorrectly and has to correct bad habits. The beginner's mind is a good, open mind.

This book is not primarily written for you if you are chiefly interested in entering bodybuilding contexts, power lifting contests, or doing Olympic lifting. You'll find some books on those topics in the Selected Bibliography and, I hope, nevertheless pick up a couple of useful tips between here and there.

This is a book for those who want to do the minimum amount of weight lifting required for physically aging as well as possible. If that's you, terrific!

10

Begin now right where you are. Seriously.

Again, I'm assuming that you are either a beginner who has never done any weight lifting or that it's at least been a long time since you've done any weightlifting.

Begin with body weight exercises. In fact, if you prefer them, they may be all you ever do or need to do! If so, I recommend Mark Lauren's YOU ARE YOUR OWN GYM [see the Selected Bibliography] and similar books. I prefer not to be limited to body weight exercises, but that may not be true for you.

If you would prefer not to be limited to them, either you'll probably have to pay to visit a commercial gym and use the equipment there or buy your own equipment to use at home. If you don't mind being limited to body weight exercises, that's fine: just use the principles in the third and fourth chapters and apply them to the body weight exercises that you select.

There are advantages and disadvantages to body weight only exercises. They require no equipment or any special location. They can all be done easily at home with only "equipment" that is likely to be there anyway (such as a towel or chair). In fact, they can be done almost anywhere. They tend to be better for increasing muscular endurance rather than muscular strength. On the other hand, they can actually take longer to do than using free weights or resistance machines. It can be good, too, if where you train is not where you usually are. Furthermore, it's easier to notice improvements as you use, say, heavier dumbbells or barbells.

If, like me, you do want to use free weights (barbells and dumbbells) or resistance machines, then that's fine as long as you have done some initial training first using your body as weight to familiarize your body with strength training..

With respect to the question whether it is better to use free weights or resistance machines, each has advantages and disadvantages. If you want to train at home, as I do, then unless you are wealthy you'll find the cost of a set of resistance machines and the space they require prohibitive. They take up a lot of room and any good set will cost tens of thousands of dollars. So, unless you are wealthy, if you prefer resistance machines to free weights, you'll need to visit someone else's gym – which is not necessarily bad. It's possible to get a good workout using either free weights or resistance machines.

With respect to the question whether it's better to train in a home gym or in a commercial gym, each has advantages and disadvantages.

A commercial gym is likely to have a wider variety of equipment. It can be a good place to find a good training partner and some helpful instruction. It can have a good atmosphere for training, too. On the other hand, you'll have to pay a monthly or yearly fee and travel to it. You may have to train only at certain times and, when you do, you may have to wait in line to use certain equipment or machines. You may be surrounded by clueless trainees who look at you strangely when you are training properly, in other words, intensely. (It's happened to me and it's uncomfortable.) Having other trainees around can also be distracting. When I occasionally use a commercial gym when I'm away from home, I find it very distracting to notice other trainees either doing dangerous exercises or using improper exercise technique on normally safe exercises. I always have to decide whether or not I should say something and, if so, what's the most helpful way to say it—and that's not what I want to be thinking about when training.

I'm not financially wealthy. I prefer not to pay monthly or yearly fees to a commercial gym. Yes, I mostly must train without using lots of different resistance machines, but that's only a minor disadvantage. Over the years, I have built up what I consider to be a nicely equipped home gym. I have "practice" dumbbells and barbells as well as "Olympic" dumbbells and barbells. I have a power rack and two different benches. I have a lat pulldown machine, a seated calf machine, a back raise machine, a leg raise machine, and used to have an angled leg press machine. I have specialty bars (for example, both practice and Olympic e-z curl bars, a trap bar, a safety-squat bar, and a forearm lever bar) and some specialty equipment (for example, grippers). I've plenty minor accoutrements, too.

Yes, I had to purchase all that equipment and I spent thousands of dollars doing so. However, good equipment never wears out or goes out of style. I actually still use some equipment that I first purchased when I was in high school over 60 years ago! Well-chosen weight lifting equipment can be a very good investment.

I have also had the great advantage of living in the same place for over 40 years and having sufficient room for a relatively well-equipped home gym. Since I live many miles from even the nearest commercial facility, using my home gym is especially convenient. It's private. The only distractions, such as music, are ones that I prefer. I control its temperature and humidity. Since there's only my longtime training partner there with me, it's easy to leave my ego at the door. Maintaining the equipment and keeping it clean is easy.

Still, I did have to purchase it all and to house it all these years. Most of the time the space occupied by my gym is unused for anything else. While not meeting anyone during training is an advantage for me, it might not be for you. Furthermore, even if you want your own home gym, it's best initially to use someone else's equipment just to figure out exactly what you want to purchase for your home gym and what order to make your purchases.

What about the issue of whether it's better to have a training partner or to train alone?

The answer depends upon you and upon the training partner.

Some people simply prefer training alone. They benefit from being single-mindedly focused on what they are doing. If that's you, there's no problem training alone as long as you understand what you are doing and have the proper equipment. For example, if you don't know what you are doing and don't have the proper equipment, it's actually possibly to kill yourself weight lifting. I've heard that, on average, several trainees each year in North America kill themselves. The most common way is that, while doing bench presses outside a power rack without properly set safety bars and without a spotter, they pass out because they are breathing incorrectly and the heavy barbell falls on their throats. If you kill yourself that way after reading this book, shame on you! You failed to pay attention.

The chief reason why it's helpful to have a good training partner is to help you overcome the inertia of doing nothing. Weightlifting is brutally hard work. It requires real effort to train intensely. If you don't train intensely, don't bother. If, like me, you are physically lazy, it's really helpful to have a reliable training partner who shows up regularly, on time, ready to train. When my partner shows up, I simply must get going. It's time to drop my excuses and get moving some poundages.

On the other hand, having a poor training partner is counter-productive. Just as it's better to live alone than with a partner with whom you don't get along, it's better to train alone than to have a poor training partner. A poor training partner is one who is unreliable, has a poor attitude about training, fails to encourage you, or fails to train hard.

A good training partner will also be helpful as a spotter on certain exercises and for noticing less-than-perfect exercise technique when you tire and your form gets sloppy. He or she may also keep learning about weight lifting and, so, contribute understanding to the hobby that you are engaged in together.

Again, improving the strength of your muscles, connective tissues, and bones is a key component with respect to aging as well as possible physically. Here's a related fact that may surprise you: weightlifting has powerful psychological benefits! I'm not sure why it does, but it does. If you don't already understand that from personal experience, I encourage you to find that out for yourself.

Perhaps at least part of the explanation is that, since weight lifting has so many positive physical benefits, we naturally want to maximize them. It's good to feel strong and to be strong! (I love it when, occasionally, something happens, I react physically, and someone remarks how strong I am. That's actually happened more than once, probably because I'm a "sleeper" in the sense that I don't look as strong as I am.) The point is that being stronger seems naturally to lead to other good physical habits such as eating well and getting plenty of sleep and recovery. If you are exercising well, eating well, and sleeping well, you are going to be feeling about as good physically all day long as it's possible to feel. This may account for at least some of its psychological benefits.

Another part of the explanation is that moving relatively heavy weight requires single-minded focus, which always dispels compulsive thoughts. As I have argued elsewhere, compulsive thoughts obstruct us from living well. When we drop them by becoming what we are doing, we enter the zone that is free of time, self, and other unnecessary thoughts. In other words, actually training hard can be an optimal or flow experience.

As some wag asked, if you don't take care of your body, where else are you going to live?

If you have never lifted weights and begin by following the suggestions in this book, you may be on the verge of a real breakthrough. <u>You may be about to begin to feel better physically than you have ever felt in your life!</u>

Weightlifting effectively means doing things that get you closer to your goal (and avoiding doing things that take you farther from your goal).

Let's consider here four aspects of weightlifting effectively, namely, training in relation to your other activities, the best kinds of exercises to use, the most effective way of using those exercises, and how to avoid overtraining.

First, obviously when you train relates to your other physical activities such as sleeping and eating.

With respect to sleeping, if you are tired for some reason, don't train. Wait a day until you are more refreshed. This is an example of an important principle: *pay attention to your body.* Instead of training on some artificial schedule, notice the condition of your body and don't train when you are injured, ill, tired, or just really "off."

For most people, the best training times seem to be late mornings and late afternoons. (My training partner and I almost always start warming up at 11:00 a.m.)

If you follow my recommendations, you'll be training only once or twice weekly. That's sufficient if you are training properly. Sometimes, some people (especially eager young male beginners who think that in just a few months they'll look like Arnold Schwarzenegger or Ronnie Coleman in their primes) train frequently as well as hard based on the false assumption that we grow in the gym.

No, we grow outside the gym. What we do in the gym is stimulate growth. It also takes proper nutrition, sleep, and recovery to foster growth. If you train too frequently, as many a young man has discovered to his dismay, you'll actually get weaker! (I return to this when I cover overtraining later in this chapter.)

Drink plenty of clean water.

So get plenty of sleep and rest. There's nothing wrong with the usual 8 hours of sleep nightly. In terms of other physical activities, minimize them with one exception: once or twice weekly it's good to get some intense (hence, brief) fitness exercise. For example, do high intensity interval training for 10 or 15 minutes twice weekly in addition to your one or two weightlifting sessions that are less than 10 minutes each. Even then, you may want to do only one weight lifting session, for a total of just 3 brief workouts weekly with a full rest day between each workout.

In terms of eating prior to training, eat a good meal sometime in the four hours just prior to a weightlifting workout and do not eat in the 90-minute period just before a weightlifting workout. Experiment and find the timing that works best for you. (Eating no closer than two hours before training works well for me.)

In terms of eating after training, it's important to maximize the anabolic window created by proper weight training by having a well-designed protein shake within 15 minutes after you finish a weightlifting workout.

Second, what kind of exercises should you do?

The first rule of exercising is: *don't make things worse.* You are likely to make things worse if you select dangerous exercises or use improper exercise technique on generally safe exercises.

You won't find any dangerous exercises recommended in this book. It's surprising how many common exercises are dangerous, including behind-the-neck pulldowns, behind-the neck presses, and Smith machine squats. They are particularly insidious because, while many people do them for years without any problems, eventually they wind up with serious shoulder or knee problems because of them. (I never had any difficulty doing behind-the-neck barbell presses, for example, but I gave them up for good once I realized that our shoulders are not properly structured for doing them. Despite being nearly 80 and training intensely for many years, I don't have any shoulder problems. Partly that's genetic luck, but partly it's because I have never done much to abuse them.) Done properly, weightlifting is safe.

Even if the exercises recommended in this book are safe, how can you tell what other exercises to do as you go on to intermediate training? With one exception, unless you are a master trainee, don't do any exercise that isn't found in Stuart McRobert's book *BUILD MUSCLE LOSE FAT LOOK GREAT.* The one exception is his version of weighted dips. In fact, dips are an excellent exercise and weighted dips can be extremely productive. However, if you do them, do not hang the weight off your waist; instead, hang it around your neck (using, perhaps, a chain wrapped in a towel). If you think about it for just a moment, by doing dips with weights hanging off your waist and dangling between your knees, you are using that weight to pull your spine apart! I had a friend who was a former Mr. Ohio bodybuilder who used to use 300 lbs. doing weighted chins that way, and he wound up spending six months lying in bed recovering from a back injury. (I did write McRobert about that; he agreed with me and wrote back telling me he'd change his book in its next edition, but he failed to make the change.)

One reason I like *BUILD MUSCLE LOSE FAT LOOK GREAT* is his emphasis on safety. With that one exception, you may select any exercise in that book and, as long as you do it as he or I teach, you'll be fine.

In terms of the kinds of exercises you should do, there are three chief points. First, use perfect exercise technique on every rep even if you are using a generally safe exercise. Pay attention to form, especially when you are tired. Second, never do dangerous exercises. Third, focus on doing compound exercises. What are they and why are they the best exercises?

Compound exercises are multi-joint exercises. By way of contrast, isolation exercises involve just one joint.

All exercises involve opposing muscle groups. For example, suppose that you are standing up and your arm is hanging at your side. If you keep your elbow pointed towards the ground while you raise your hand to your shoulder, you have used your biceps to curl your lower arm. Now, while keeping your hand touching your shoulder, point your elbow towards the sky and then straighten your hand towards the sky. You'll use your triceps to straighten your arm. So the biceps and triceps create motion in the lower arm by being attached by tendons to the appropriate bones. When the agonist muscle group contracts, the bone moves one way; when the antagonist muscle group contracts, the bone moves the other way.

An elbow is one joint. It's possible to train biceps and triceps by using isolation exercises. They are perfectly good exercises.

However, compound exercises involve multiple joints and, therefore, multiple muscle groups. This means that you get more benefit in terms of improved muscle tissue, connective tissue, and bony tissue for your exertion than it's possible to get with isolation exercises. Since training energy is limited, it's generally better to focus on compound rather than isolation exercises.

The best compound exercises are *squats, deadlifts, dips, presses, rows, and chins* (or pull-downs). Each one of them has multiple variations. Just using compound exercises you'll never run out of productive combinations.

This doesn't mean, however, that it's always best to avoid isolation exercises. It's not. Sometimes it's important to work on promoting balance by bringing up a lagging muscle group. Ever notice how many athletes have hamstring problems? Your risk of injury increases unless you promote muscular balance. If, as is popular, you focus on building up your thighs and never seriously train your hamstrings using isolation exercises, you are creating a strength imbalance and, so, setting yourself up for a preventable injury.

Furthermore, sometimes isolation exercises target stabilizing muscles that are strengthened to prevent injury. For example, you may want a stronger grip and do isolation exercises for the forearms. You may want to do D.A.R.D. raises to strengthen the shin muscles if you do calf raises. Not all exercises that target stabilizing muscles, though, are isolation (for example, side bends).

This discussion gives you a peek at just how interesting designing an excellent training routine can be. As a beginner, though, you should not be designing your own routines. The chief point here is simply to realize that you should mostly be doing compound exercises rather than isolation exercises.

Third, what's the most effective way of performing exercises?

The answer is to focus on finding and using the "sweet spot" on different compound exercises. By way of contrast, it is not to focus on always doing a full range of motion.

For example, think of a standing barbell curl. Instead of imagining curling one arm as we just did, let's imagine curling both arms simultaneously. You are standing upright and gripping a barbell in your hands, which are just in front of your thighs. Without moving anything else, curl the barbell to your clavicles. Notice how, near the top of the movement, the barbell just fell in towards your clavicles. While it was falling in, there was no tension on your biceps, which is what you are trying to train doing the curls in the first place. In other words, the top part of the range of motion of that exercise is useless in terms of working your biceps! The solution is simple: don't do things like that.

Similarly, imagine doing a back squat and then standing up again. Once you are all the way up and your knees are locked, you are resting! You certainly aren't working any muscle groups (other than secondary stabilizing muscle groups). Therefore, when you squat, don't stand all the way up until you are done exercising.

Similarly, imagine doing deadlifts and, between repetitions, letting the plates of the barbell rest on the floor. What good is that? It's not. Instead, just lightly and briefly touch the plates to the floor (without ever bouncing them off the floor) and ascend.

I'm not saying that a full range of motion is always counterproductive. It's not. For some exercises, for example, seated dumbbell presses, it's fine at least until the arm or arms are locked at the top. The reason is that the tension is not taken off the targeted muscle groups throughout the whole range of motion. Finding the sweet spot means using the range of motion that does not remove maximum tension from the targeted muscle groups.

So, the key is the time per repetition that the target muscle group is under tension, which is also known as "time under load" abbreviated 'TUL'. Once you begin a set of exercises, move only in the sweet spot of the possible range of motion until you have completed the set.

What's the best TUL? It's between about 40 and 90 seconds. Anything under about 35 seconds and you are not stimulating the target muscle group sufficiently. Anything over about 90 seconds is stimulating it too much.

This has direct training implications. In general, use only the sweet spot of various compound exercises and ensure that the total TUL for each exercise is not less than 40 seconds and not more than 90 seconds.

Suppose you were doing, for example, 3 sets of 5 repetitions on deadlifts. If each rep took 4 seconds, that would be a TUL for each set of 20 seconds (5 x 4) and a total TUL for the exercise of 60 seconds (3 x 20). Since 60 is between 40 and 90, that's fine.

Here's my question: why do three sets? It's unnecessary for beginners to do multiple sets. (Doing them can be a useful training tactic for intermediate and advanced trainees.) If so, why not just do 1 set such that its TUL is between 40 and 90?

That's what I recommend in this book. So, if you were doing deadlifts, you would begin moving the bar and keep it moving for at least 40 seconds and for at most 90 seconds.

String 5 such compound exercises together and you'll be able to get a terrific workout in under 10 minutes!

Here's why: each of the five exercises will last a maximum of 90 seconds. That's 7 ½ minutes. If it takes you a total of 2 minutes total transition time to move from each exercise to the next, that's a workout in 9 ½ minutes!

If you're able to set up the exercises in advance (which is easier in a home gym than in a crowded commercial gym), most of the exercises won't take the full 90 seconds. Let's suppose that they average 60 seconds. Well, that's three minutes of exercise time plus however long it takes you to move from one exercise to the next—probably 2 or 3 minutes total. If you spend three minutes exercising and three minutes transitioning, that's a total workout in just 6 minutes on the clock!

You do have time for that once or twice a week, don't you?

Fourth, what's the best way of avoiding overtraining?

It's simply to pay attention to your body.

Suppose you have not been lifting weights and begin a weightlifting routine. For a day or two afterwards, you may experience DOMS [delayed onset muscular soreness]. That occurs as your body is growing stronger by repairing the stress you caused it in the gym.

Here's the rule to avoid overtraining: <u>To ensure both systemic as well as localized recovery, wait at least 24 to 48 hours after all DOMS has disappeared before lifting weights again</u>. Make no exceptions to that rule.

That will ensure that you are recovering sufficiently. It also helps, of course, to eat well, which means eating plenty of proteins and fats from natural sources, and to drink well, which means drinking at least 2 or 3 quarts of clean water daily.

Overtraining is a result of misusing your body. Think of it as a stop signal from your body that it's foolish to ignore. Since it's a very common problem among strength athletes, please become an expert in avoiding overtraining. How? Whenever you sense it, back off. The rule is simple: <u>whenever you are in doubt, rest too much rather than too little</u>.

How can you tell if you may be overtrained? Its symptoms include: frequent colds; frequent minor injuries; persistent soreness and stiffness in muscles, joints, or tendons; loss of enthusiasm for exercising; inability to relax; sleep problems; loss of appetite; headaches; and a decrease in intellectual or academic work or performance.

Is your life balanced? Overtraining is most common among trainees who become attached to exercising. The purpose of exercise is to enhance life. As I have argued elsewhere, the truth is that it is not necessary at all to exercise physically to live well.

Your ability to recover from exercise is limited. Too much exercise can be worse that too little. Though very beneficial, intense exercise (whether it's fitness exercise or weightlifting) stresses your internal organs like your kidneys, your liver, and your pancreas. It's important always to let them recover fully from exercising. So, if you learn to pay attention to your body, you'll be able to determine a balance of fitness exercise, weight lifting, and rest and recovery that works well for you.

If two brief weight lifting workouts and two brief fitness workouts weekly are too much, do less. Try one brief weight lifting workout and two brief fitness workouts weekly. That can be less than 30 minutes weekly of well-spaced exercise and, if you are normally healthy, eating well, and otherwise getting sufficient rest and recovery, it's very unlikely that you will suffer from overtraining.

4: Training Efficiently

Weight lifting efficiently means performing tasks as economically as possible so that you get the most benefit from the least exertion.

In this chapter you'll find seven principles for ensuring that you are lifting weights efficiently (in no particular order).

First, **warm up**. What does that mean specifically?

It means elevating your heart rate, lubricating your joints, and getting your major muscle groups warm. How?

A good warm up has two parts: general and specific.

Do a general warm up by, for example, riding on a stationary bike for 5 minutes with gradually increasing intensity before doing anything else.

Then do some moving stretches to warm up your joints. For example, stand with your feet about shoulder width apart. With your arms straight out horizontally to the sides with elbows locked and palms towards the floor, begin by making small circles in the air with your arms and gradually increase the size of those circles. Then, with your palms facing away from the floor, rotate them the other way in gradually increasing circles. Rotate your torso, legs, and feet similarly. Do a bit of gentle stretching for your calves, Achilles tendons, thighs, and neck.

The purpose of this kind of warm up is not to increase flexibility. If you want to do that, use static stretching after your workouts once or twice weekly.

After you've completed the general warm-up, do some specific warm ups for the exercises that you'll be doing during training. The purpose of specific warm-ups is to increase the amount of blood in the muscles and connective tissues that you'll be using while performing the exercises that make up your weight lifting workout.

There is no one best way to do specific warm-ups. In general, use a lighter weight than you'll use during your work sets and do a few more reps than you'd normally do during your work sets. It's a balancing act: it's important to get sufficiently warmed up without doing so much work that your performance on works sets is undermined.

For example, suppose that you are going to use a 100 pound barbell for incline presses during your work set. For a specific warm up, try a 60 pound barbell and do 5 reps using a full range of motion and immediately do 5 more reps in the sweet spot, which is in the lower two-thirds of the range of motion. Rest a minute. Then take an 80 pound barbell and do 3 full range reps followed immediately by 3 reps in the sweet spot. Then you should be ready to go; the relevant muscle groups and connective tissues should be primed for some heavy work.

For the program suggested in this book, do all your warmups before you begin your first work set for the first exercise. You do not need to do specific warmups for each of the five exercises if you have already used a muscle group in a previous warm up. For example, if you have already warmed up for flat bench presses, you do not then need to warm up for seated dumbbell presses because your pectorals, triceps, and deltoids will already be warmed up.

I believe that warming up this way reduces the chance of injury. The older you are, the more important it is to warm up thoroughly.

Second, **always use perfect exercise technique**.

It's often the little details that matter. If your elbows are in the wrong position or your hand spacing is incorrect, you may injure yourself. With respect to the exercises described later in this book, pay attention to all the apparently minor details.

Perform every repetition smoothly and slowly without momentum. If you ever find yourself twisting, bouncing, swinging, squirming, or distorting your body in unusual ways, stop immediately and lower the weight you are using. Always control descents, too; never just let the weight drop.

<u>Maintain tension on the targeted muscle group throughout the exercise without using momentum.</u>

Focus on what you are doing. Imagine the target muscle engorging with oxygenated blood and growing larger and stronger. Imagine your tendons and ligaments thickening and becoming stronger. Make use of the mind.

On both upper and lower body exercises, keep your back in the power position, in other words, with your lower back slightly concave and your stomach pushed out. Maintain excellent posture.

On work sets, stay within the sweet spot so that you are constantly maintaining the tension. Typically, it's the bottom half of the range of motion that is critical.

However, even if the exercises that you use are not generally dangerous and even if you are doing them with perfect exercise technique, it doesn't follow that a specific exercise will work well for you. That's why it's important to begin with relatively light weights (such as your body weight) so that, if you have a problem with a specific exercise, it won't be a serious problem.

Third, **change your routine at least every three months**.

Our bodies are wonderfully adaptable. After a few weeks, as your body adapts to whatever routine you are using, that routine will become less productive. So here's what to do: after 7 or 11 weeks of training, deliberately do no weight lifting at all for one full week and then resume training with a different routine or at least different exercise variations.

It's easy to come up with different routines simply by substituting different exercises or by changing the order in which you do exercises. The point is that it's very unnatural and counter-productive (unless you are foolishly using anabolic steroids) to stick to the same routine month after month.

Fourth, **start each workout with the most productive exercise**.

Since the energy you have for training is limited, this makes intuitive sense. In practice it means always starting with some variation of either squats or deadlifts. Give them all you have! Since they provide the maximum return, really hit them hard. Remember, though, on them always keep one rep or a little time in you. If you go to failure on squats or deadlifts, you increase your chances of injury – and injuries retard progress.

Fifth, **train progressively**.

Each workout try your best to do at least a little better on each exercise. In other words, try to train for a few more seconds or with slightly more weight. You won't always be able to do that; you will have days when it's impossible for whatever reason. Just resolve each time to work as hard as you are able to work to do that.

For example, suppose that your first exercise is squats and, last time, you quit after 52 seconds using 185 lbs. Next time, go for 55 or 60 seconds. That's slightly harder. That's what it means to train progressively.

Sixth, **make exercises more difficult**.

This one seems counter-intuitive. If you let it, your body will always try to move the weight with the least energy expenditure possible. If you let it, it will always want to use momentum and to use sloppy technique by using other muscle groups to assist the ones you are training.

So look for ways to counter this natural tendency. Why? By making exercises more difficult, you'll be able to get the same results using less weight. By using less weight, you'll automatically reduce the chances of injury.

For example, go into any commercial gym and watch how fast people are training. You may see someone doing bench presses doing one rep every 3 seconds. Wrong! You may see someone bouncing the bar off his chest at the bottom of a bench press. Wrong! If you see anyone doing squats, you may see that person bouncing at the bottom of a squat to get some upward momentum going. Wrong!

Use less weight. Slow down rep speed. Don't cheat.

Seven, **deliberately strengthen stabilizing muscles**.

Since this is less important for beginners than for intermediate or advanced trainees, I don't otherwise make a point of it in this book.

Still, it's definitely an idea that, when executed, decreases the chances of injury. The stabilizing muscles are the secondary muscles that assist an exercise's targeted primary muscles. At the end of workouts, it's always a good idea to do some grip exercises or side bends or abdominal work. It the long run, they can really become important. However, if you are a beginner, there's no need to worry about them for a few months.

On the other hand, even if you are a beginner, you may be aware of lagging muscle groups. If so and if you want to do a little special work on them, just do it at the end of your workouts.

30

5: Initial routines

Before you begin using the weight lifting routines provided in this chapter, it's important to begin with body weight exercises. So, after I offer desciptions of how to do some basic body weight exercises, you'll find the initial routines. In the following chapters, you'll find detailed descriptions of how to perform the weight lifting exercises correctly using free weights.

(If you only happen to have access to resistance machines, you'll need to substitute resistance machine exercises for the free weight exercises. There are many, many different kinds of resistance machines. Presumably, you are using them because they happen to be in a commercial gym you are using. You should be able to get training from the gym's staff on how to use those machines correctly. Just use the techniques you learn from them in accordance with the principles discussed in the previous two chapters.)

Body Weight Exercises:

For more detailed exercise descriptions of body weight exercises, I recommend *YOU ARE YOUR OWN GYM*.

AIR SQUATS: Stand with your feet about shoulder width apart with your toes pointing outwards at about a 45 degree angle. As you bend your knees, have them track in the direction that your toes are pointing and raise your arms straight in front of you for balance. Your upper body will learn a bit forward as you descend. Keep your arms crossed on your chest or your hands on your hips. Keep your knees behind your toes; in other words, sit back as you descend. Keep the weight on your heels. When your butt gets a couple of inches from the floor, use your thighs to lift yourself up again.

Do not straighten your legs at the top or you'll be resting. Instead, when the tension on your thighs begins decreasing significantly, begin another descent.

As always, and I won't repeat this for each exercise, each rep should take about 10 or 15 seconds. Continue for at least 40 seconds.

GOOD MORNINGS: Stand with your feet about shoulder width apart. Clasp your hands behind your head. Bow down forward keeping your back arched (with chest and butt out) and your legs almost straight but unlocked. Return to the starting position.

PUSH UPS. Lie on your stomach with your legs together, your hands under your shoulders, and the underside of your toes on the floor. While keeping your body straight, push yourself up until your arms are nearly straight. Lower until your chest lightly touches the ground and, without resting on the floor, repeat.

If you are too weak to do push ups, you may begin by doing wall push ups. Then do them while keeping your knees on the floor.

SEATED DIPS. Find a stable horizontal surface such as a hard chair or a bench that is thigh high. Facing away from it, put your palms on the edge closest to your butt with your knuckles pointing forward. Walk your legs forward until they are straight out in front of you with your heels resting on the floor and your butt a couple of inches in front of the surface. While bending only at the shoulders and elbows and keeping your forearms perpendicular to the floor, lower your body down until your triceps are parallel to the floor. Keep your back a couple of inches in front of the surface. Using your triceps, push yourself up again.

DIPS: Find two stable surfaces that are strong and the same height. (Parallel bars are ideal, but the tops of two strong hard chairs can work if you bend your knees.) Put the surfaces slightly wider than hip width apart. Put a palm on each surface with your arms straight. While bending only at the shoulders and elbows, lower your body down until your triceps are parallel to the floor. Push yourself back up again. Keep the motion as natural as possible.

STANDING PRESS: Find a relatively heavy item such as a loaded book box or a loaded backpack. Standing with your feet shoulder width apart, hold that item with your hands in front of your clavicles. Keeping your stomach muscles tight and your lower back concave, press the item overhead until your arms are nearly extended and then lower it.

LET ME UPS: Put a heavy dowel (and even a strong broom stick may work) about waist high between two strong supports. Lie directly under it on the floor with your chest directly under the dowel. Grab the bar with your hands about shoulder width apart and, while holding the rest of your body straight and rigid, pull yourself up towards the dowel. Only the backs of yours heels will be touching the floor. Squeeze your shoulder blades together at the top and then lower slowly.

CHINS: you'll either need a strong door or a pull-up bar. Using a door, open it partway and put a towel over its top. Wedge it so that it won't swing. Place your hands on the towel and bend your knees. Pull yourself up until your chin is over the top of the door and lower yourself slowly.

If you use a pull-up bar (or a jungle gym in a park), be sure that you don't swing your body to create momentum. Go up and down slowly.

Initial Free Weight Routines:

Here are two initial routines. I recommend doing the first one for 11 weeks and then taking 1 full week off from weight lifting. Then do the second one for 11 weeks and take another full week off from weight training.

After that, you may repeat the first routine again for 11 weeks or use some other similar routine.

If you follow this procedure, you'll get off to an excellent start.

As I have explained in the previous chapters, you will only do one set of each exercise. Use a slow rep speed, which means taking 10 or 15 seconds per rep. Keep the bar moving in the sweet spot of the range of motion, which will keep tension continuously on the targeted muscle groups.

The weight that you use should allow you to keep exercising for at least 40 seconds per set and, when you are able to go for 90 seconds or more, increase the weight the next workout.

Keep breathing; do not hold your breathe. You should breathe naturally and continuously. You'll usually exhale as the weight is moving up. Deliberately increase your rate of respiration towards the end of each set.

Do not train more than twice weekly and once weekly is fine as long as you are doing two intense sessions of fitness exercise also during a week.

Do not begin using these routines until you have developed strength using your body as weight. Here are the routines:

Routine 1:

Squats. Pull-downs or chins. Seated overhead presses with thick bar. Incline dumbbell presses. Partial deadlifts using either an Olympic bar or a trap bar.

Routine 2:

Box squats. Pull downs or chins. Seated dumbbell presses. Bench presses. Sumo deadlifts.

The following chapters explain exactly how to do these exercises correctly. Again, the most important exercises are the squats and deadlifts. Please focus on mastering their techniques.

If you don't happen to have access to some piece of recommended equipment (for example, a thick bar or dumbbells), just substitute other equipment to come as close as you are able to come to the recommended exercise. Except for squats and deadlifts, there's nothing magical about the other exercises; other excellent substitutes are available that are both effective and safe.

Do not rest between exercises; move quickly from each exercise to the next. Track your time by recording beginning and ending times as well as the number of seconds for each exercise work set. Keep a written record.

6: Squats

If you have never done squats (deep knee bends), deciding whether or not to do them can be confusing. Some people claim that the squat is the king of exercises, while others say that you should never squat.

Done properly, squats are very beneficial for most people. I encourage you not to be quick to dismiss them. I offer you four variations. I explain back squats in detail; simply transfer those instructions to front squats, hip belt squats or box squats insofar as they apply. If you pay close attention to detail, it's quite likely that at least one of the variations will work well for you.

Always pay attention and think safety: **always alert, never get hurt.** Squats and deadlifts are similar in that they are both extremely productive exercises for nearly everyone. However, it's important to do them correctly.

It may seem that there's a lot to master to do squats and deadlifts correctly. That's correct. One reason weightlifting is an excellent hobby is because it's so interesting. There's a lot to learn. If you realize that in advance, just decide to be patient and learn it at your own pace. Stay humble, keep an open mind, and enjoy the process.

Also, leave your ego at the gym door. You're entering the gym to do your best; you are not entering the gym to compete with anyone else. Instead of trying to rush or force some desired result, work with your body to improve a little bit each time you train.

The general description for doing **back squats** is simple. Put a barbell on the back of your shoulders. With your feet at shoulder width apart, feet pointed outward at about a 45-degree angle, and with your belly pushed forward (so that your lower back is concave), bend your knees to lower your body. Let your knees track in the direction of your toes. Sit back and down. When the tops of your thighs go below parallel to the floor, raise yourself while keeping your head up.

Here's how to avoid getting hurt and maximizing the results:

Never bounce at the bottom of a squat. To help prevent this, when you are just below parallel, start up again. Similarly, never use momentum.

Never round your back. Keep it tightly arched throughout the movement. There should be a slight hollow in your lower back. Also, keep your upper back tight with your shoulder blades pulled back and your chest pushed out.

Never squat with a board under your heels or use shoes or boots with thick heels. This is a common mistake. Instead, increase your flexibility until you're able to squat correctly with both feet flat on the floor. It's fine to squat barefoot; otherwise, use shoes, boots, or slippers with only a minimal heel and non-slippery bottoms. It's fine to wear supportive sneakers or weightlifting shoes with high tops.

Never raise your hips from the bottom before raising the bar or move the bar forward before you move it up; otherwise, you'll lean forward too far and put too much pressure on your lower back. The taller you are, the more forward you'll naturally lean. Never raise your hips faster than your shoulders.

Never squat with your knees close together. Keep your knees separated at either a medium or a wide distance apart. Push them outwards through the movement, particularly when you are ascending.

Never squat with your toes pointed forward so that your feet are parallel to each other; instead, keep your feet pointed out at least 20 degrees and 30 or 45 degrees would be better. Keep them pointed in the same direction as your upper legs unless that happens to stress them too much.

Do not descend straight down. Instead, sit back and down almost as if you were sitting on a living room sofa.

Do not look down. Look directly forward or up from the top position and keep your eyes focused on that one spot.

Especially as you ascend, keep most of the weight on your heels. Do not keep most of the weight on the balls of your feet.

Do not pick the bar off the rack until your hips are directly under the bar. When you pick it up, take a single step back (without looking down) and set your feet properly. When you finish, shuffle your feet forward until the bar is over the pins or stand; in other words, do not walk forward by raising a foot. Before racking the bar, ensure that it is over the pins or stands and that your fingers are not in the way before bending your knees to rack it.

Do not squat using a sweaty shirt; ensure that your shirt is dry.

Consider using chalk or rosin on your hands before a work set. It's not necessary, but it can help. (Commercial gyms that don't have chalk are not designed for serious training.) You may also have someone apply it to the back top of your shirt where the bar will rest during the movement.

Never turn your head while squatting.

Never do deadlifts before doing squats.

Never squat if you have any trace of DOMS.

If you use a lifting belt, inhale before descending and push your belly hard against the inside of the belt. Exhale as you ascend.

Do not stand all the way up at the top and lock your knees. Instead, keep your back tight and your knees unlocked to keep tension on your muscles until the set is over.

Never squat in a Smith machine. The reason is that they force the bar to travel straight up and down, which is an unnatural, hence dangerous, motion. If you put your feet forward when doing Smith machine squats, you will prevent your knees from going too far forward near the bottom of the movement, but you'll also be simultaneously putting your lower back at risk. If you instead put your feet under your shoulders, you'll find as you descend that the load will shift over the balls of your feet, which will increase the pressure on your knees. In other words, using a Smith machine for squats is always dangerous.

It's a good idea to keep your knees warm while squatting. You may purchase thick rubber sleeves that you pull up over your knees to keep them warm. As long as you wash them and let them dry properly after every use, they'll last for many years. Using them won't make squatting easier. They just keep your knees warm.

Especially if you have ever had any knee trouble, you may wrap your knees with heavy elastic bandages. The more tightly you wrap them, the more support they will provide.

If you have ever had any knee problems, you may well find that squatting is very helpful. It strengthens the muscles and tendons that bend and straighten the leg and, so, helps the knees to function well.

Front squats are a great variation to back squats. Basically, you hold the barbell in front of your clavicles with your elbows keeping your upper arms parallel to the floor. You'll use a bit less weight on front squats than on back squats. They feel awkward initially, but, once you get the movement mastered, they are extremely productive.

Hip belt squats are another great variation to back squats. To do them, you'll need a hip belt which fits tightly around your hips. The barbell hangs between your knees pointed directly in front of you. Since the weight is supported by your hips rather than your upper torso, hip belt squats are a terrific alternative for anyone who has a back problem. You'll use a lot less weight on hip belt squats than on back squats. It is awkward getting into and out of position, but they will really torch your thighs even with relatively light weights. They are safer than either back squats or front squats.

There is an underused variation of full squats that seems to be safer and more effective than standard back squats, namely, **box squats**. If you want to boost your back squat poundage, do box squats for a couple of months and then return to back squats. You may be delighted at your progress.

Box squats are a terrific variation. The equipment is the same as for back squats except that you will also need a box or bench of exactly the right height for you. It may or may not be padded. Ensure that the tops of your thighs when you are seated on the box are just slightly under parallel.

Doing box squats is very similar to doing back squats. It's never a bad idea to wear a weightlifting belt when doing squats, deadlifts, or overhead presses. If you do, before descending, fill your abdomen with air and push out against the belt for the duration of the rep. Keep your back tightly arched. When descending and ascending, deliberately push your knees outward. Use a wide stance.

Here's the difference: lower yourself until the box is supporting you and the barbell for half a second or a second. Keep everything tight except for somewhat relaxing your hip flexors and glute muscles. While sitting on the box correctly, your shins will be just past perpendicular. Then ascend while keeping your head up. Try to push your traps into the bar first, followed immediately by the hips and glutes and, finally, the legs.

Do not rock on the box. Don't just touch and go off the box; actually sit on it for a moment. Except mainly for your hip flexors for a moment while you are on the box, don't fail to keep all muscle groups tight throughout the movement.

As usual, don't just sit straight down when descending; instead, sit back and down. When ascending, don't turn it into a good morning by raising your hips first. When you stand up, don't lock your knees; keep the tension on.

You won't master them without doing them a few times. Start with a relatively light weight, lighter than what you use for back squats. Assuming that you already have mastered back squats, after several workouts box squats will begin to feel very familiar and you may begin increasing your poundage. (Without chains or bands, in my late 60s I was doing sets of about 10 reps with 230 pounds after about my third time doing them.)

You may prefer box squats so much to regular back squats that you may be reluctant to use back squats ever again. If so, don't go back to them.

(I learned about box squats from Louie Simmons of Westside barbell. There are free YouTube videos of him and other power lifters doing box squats in training.)

There are four great ways to squat. Pick one, master it, and eventually try the other three as well. Almost certainly, you'll find one that is very productive for you.

In fact, don't be surprised if you develop a love/hate relationship with them! You may love their benefits but hate doing them. The intensity required to do them well is, remember, also psychologically as well as physically beneficial. When you are squatting with a weight that is heavy for you, you will be paying attention to the present moment. You will not be lost elsewhere in thought.

You will, in fact, be living deeply in the present moment.

40

7. Deadlifts

If squats are not the king of weight lifting exercises, deadlifts are. There are three kinds using a barbell, namely, regular (bent-legged) deadlifts, sumo deadlifts, and partial deadlifts. There's fourth kind that is very similar except that it uses a trap bar (and they can also be done using heavy dumbbells). Each is extremely productive exercise. I encourage you to try them all.

If you follow the two routines I suggest in this book, you'll end each workout doing some kind of deadlift. They are a great complement to squats. If you do both squats and deadlifts at the same workout, always do deadlifts after doing squats. The reason is that they stress your back more and, if you do squats after already exhausting your back, you greatly increase the chances of injury.

Deadlifts are very natural. What could be more natural than picking a weight off the ground and standing up with it? Except that the weight is a barbell, that's all a deadlift is. I think they are the greatest single weightlifting exercise.

Please don't go too low with deadlifts. If you are using a common Olympic bar, ensure that there is at least a 45 pound plate on each side. When the plate touches the ground, it will automatically prevent you from going too low. At first, you may not be strong enough to use that much weight. That's not a problem: just do deadlifts inside a power rack with the safety bars put on the lowest setting. Start with an empty bar and work your way up progressively.

There's not necessarily anything wrong with doing deadlifts off the lowest bar settings in a power rack. Only powerlifters in competitions need to lift off the floor. It's not only safer, but it's also easier to load the bar.

It's important to have nonslip footwear with minimal heel height and sole thickness. Ensure that the floor isn't too slick with, say, paint or humidity. It's best to deadlift on rubber matting or a special platform built of commercial carpet on solid plywood.

Just as with squats, keep the weight mostly on your heels rather than on the balls of your feet. Do not have the stress on your toes. Keep your knees pressed outward rather than coming inward as you ascend.

The bar should be close to your shins so that it brushes against the fronts of your legs when it's moving.

Think of your arms as just links to the bar. Do not bend them; keep them straight. They will be close to vertical throughout the movement.

Keep your palms facing you, evenly spaced on the bar. Once the barbell becomes heavy enough that you feel your grip weaken, either strengthen your grip by regularly doing grip exercises, which is the best option, or resort to using wrist straps or hooks. A bar that slips out of control is dangerous. (Power lifters often use reverse grips, but that stresses the torso asymmetrically, which requires that the hands be shifted appropriately. Beginners should just keep their palms facing them.) Grip the bar with even spacing. It's a good idea to use some tape, paint, or hose around the bar to mark where you should grip.

Each foot should be evenly spaced as well. The bar will always remain parallel to a line drawn across the lifter's toes.

Begin at the bottom position with your hips a lot lower than your shoulders. As with squats, always keep your head and eyes up. Keep a tight back throughout the movement with your back in the power position (such that your lower back is slightly concave).

Shrug your shoulders vertically against the bar when you are ready to begin. As you ascend, lift simultaneously with your back and legs: push upward with your legs while simultaneously pulling with your back. If you lift primarily with either your back or your legs, you are lifting improperly. Do not rock or jerk the bar off the floor; instead, squeeze it off the floor.

For some reason unknown to me, it really helps not to think of yourself as lifting the bar at all! Instead, think of yourself as pushing the earth away from under the bar.

As you descend, ensure that your shoulders are pulled back and your shoulder blades are retracted. Never round your back. Keep your chest pushed up and out.

At the top, do not lead back and do not just stand there resting. Keep the tension on.

Move slowly: it should take about 10 or 15 seconds per rep. Never round your lower back or lean too far forward. If the bar gets out of groove, just dump it.

Never turn your head while deadlifting.

Always deadlift using collars on the bar. If a plate slips a bit, you could get injured.

Never bounce the plates off the floor; if you are using a power rack, never bound the bar off the safety bars. Lightly touch both sides to the floor and immediately ascend. Alternatively, do, say, 5 singles one after the other instead of 1 set of 5 reps.

As with squats, always keep 1 rep or some time in you. Do not go to failure. Don't employ intensity techniques such as forced reps or negative-only reps with deadlifts. As with squats, really focus to do each rep with perfect technique.

Partial deadlifts are a great complement to squats. They are sometimes called "stiff-legged" deadlifts, but that name is misleading because it is important not to keep your knees locked while doing them. Sometimes they are also called "Romanian" deadlifts. Keep your legs generally straight but unlocked.

The main difference between partial and regular deadlifts is that the range of motion on partial deadlifts is decreased. Always do them in a power rack with the safety bars set so that when the barbell is resting on the safety bars it is somewhat below your kneecaps with your knees slightly bent. What this will do is to minimize how much your thighs are involved while still enabling you to work your back, glutes, and hamstrings hard.

Your knees should straighten naturally as you ascend and then bend again slightly during the descent. Of course, when doing a multiple rep set, do not rest the barbell on the safety bars at the bottom; just touch them lightly and ascend. In other words, don't bounce the bar off the safety bars.

Exhale either at the top or as you ascend. You may inhale as you descend or inhale at the top and hold it as you ascend.

Never do full range of motion partial deadlifts. (Sometimes foolish trainees will do them standing on the end of a bench so that they can lower their hands all the way to the tops of their feet. Yikes!)

You may do partial deadlifts using a **trap bar** instead of a barbell. In fact, if you have access to a trap bar, I suggest that you make this the first kind of deadlift to master. However, since a trap bar is insufficiently wide to be able to use the safety bars in a power rack, you'll need to find boxes of a suitable height to use under its plates.

Especially if you are over six feet tall, you may come to prefer **sumo deadlifts** to regular deadlifts because they will improve your leverage. If you find that they work better for you (and they do for me, probably because I'm 6'2"), you may always substitute sumo deadlifts for regular deadlifts.

Although sumo deadlifts and regular deadlifts look radically different, they are actually quite similar. Usually the torso does not tip quite as far forward when doing sumo deadlifts compared to regular deadlifts.

Use a stance that is moderately wide. If you are tall, your toes may nearly be as wide as the insides of the plates on the barbell. Again, your toes should be pointed out at about a 45 degree angle or slightly less.

As you descend to grip the bar, you'll keep your hands inside your knees and grip the bar at about hip width. (If you are gripping the bar on the smooth section in its center, your hands are too close together and you'll find it more difficult to balance the bar during movement.)

The movement is very similar to that of a regular deadlift. You may find that your knees are less of an obstacle to get over because of the wider stance. That's why you may bend forward less than when doing a regular deadlift.

Build up the poundage you are using slowly and progressively. You may want to alternate between doing regular deadlifts for a couple of months and then doing sumo deadlifts for a couple of months until you are confident about which style works best for you. Once you determine that, just keep using that style and forget using the other style.

Deadlifts are a great exercise. I hope that you master them and are able to train well using them until your dotage.

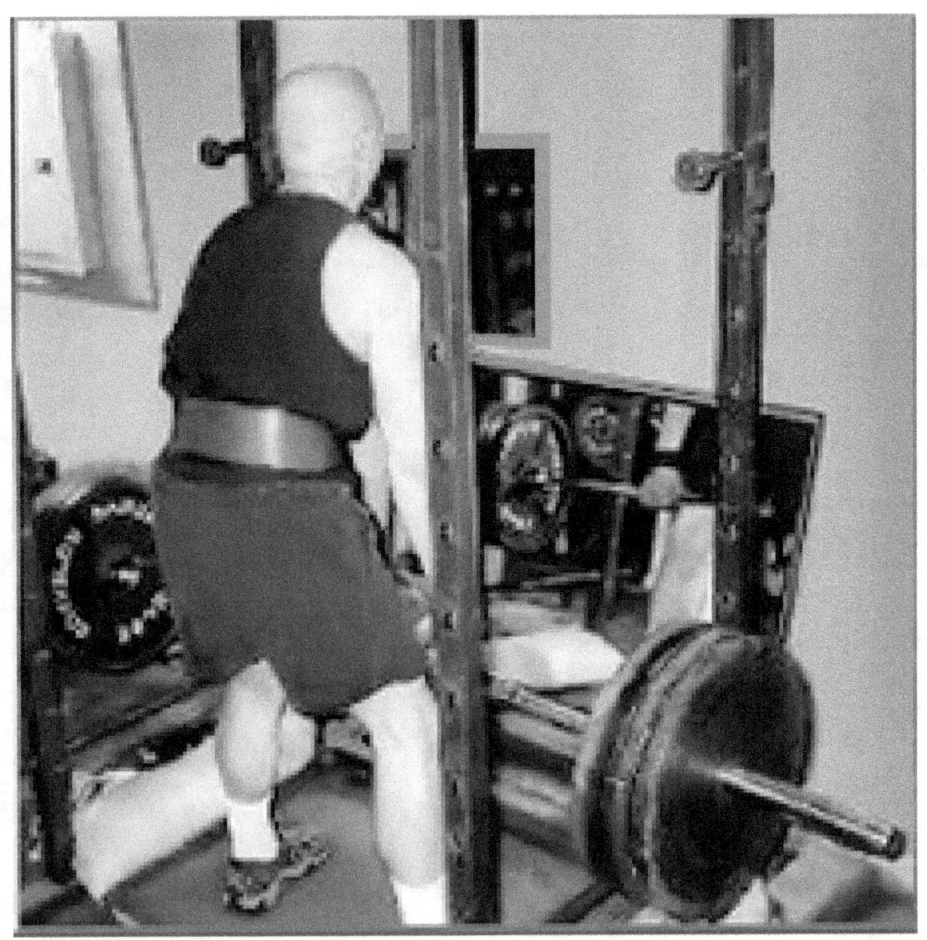

That's a photo of me in my home gym in front of a mirror (to ensure the bar was level) when I was in my 60s doing partial deadlifts for reps with 405 pounds.

8. Bench presses

For most trainees the bench press is a very good upper body exercise.

Perhaps because it's done lying flat on your back, it's certainly a popular exercise. Although it's more important to master squats or deadlifts, "How much can you bench?" is a more popular question than either "How much can you squat?" or "How much can you deadlift?"

It's a more productive exercise for some than for others. Differences in individual body structure matter a lot when benching. For example, long arms are a real disadvantage.

Regardless of your natural leverage, if you use proper exercise technique and some auxiliary exercises, your pectorals, deltoids, triceps, and upper back muscles will really benefit.

Either master perfect barbell bench press technique or don't do them.

The reason for this is simple: again, they are the most deadly weight lifting exercise. If you mess up your technique on other exercises, you might strain or sprain or even break something or blow out a joint. If you drop a loaded barbell onto your throat when doing a barbell bench press, you could kill yourself. Sadly and unnecessarily, many have.

There's more to mastering barbell bench press technique that you might initially think.

If you are a beginner, if you are breathing correctly during the exercise and a day or two afterwards experiencing some DOMS in your pectorals, you are doing alright. The initial task is to master barbell bench press technique sufficiently well so that you do them safely and also avoid becoming a shoulder bench presser.

If you don't have spotters, *only* do benches inside a power rack with properly positioned safety bars (or something similar like squat stands or a half rack).

Use a horizontal bench with a straight barbell. Center the bench between the weight supports so that (i) you won't hit them when moving the bar up or down and (ii) you minimize how far you have to move the bar horizontally when racking or unracking it.

When racked the bar may be directly above your nose or forehead – it depends upon what works best for you. The safety bars should be set so that they are about one inch below your inflated chest when you are in position. Use an unloaded bar to ensure that everything is adjusted properly.

Lie back on the bench under the bar with your feet flat on the floor and wider than your shoulders. Your heels should be directly under your knees; do not bring them closer to your head or you will tend to arch your back too much. Do not lift your heels off the floor when doing a barbell bench press or otherwise squirm around.

Grip width is important. Ensure that your hands are exactly equidistant from the center of the bar. How wide is the correct grip?

When you lower the empty bar to your lower pecs, have someone ensure that your forearms are vertical when viewed both from the side and from your feet; in other words, your elbows should be directly under your wrists.

Remember that hand position and always use it. It's very important to have grip consistency. You may deliberately want to vary the distance between your thumbs, but don't vary it simply because you are being inconsistent. Keep a record.

Never use a grip that is too wide. Why? It's important always to think long term in the gym, which is why you should always leave your ego at the door; a wider grip is more likely to cause shoulder or pec problems over time.

Adult men may start with a grip that is 18" between the hands and adjust it from there. Adult women may start with a grip that is 14".

Use whichever grip you prefer. You'll probably want to wrap your thumbs under and around the bar like powerlifters always do. On the other hand, a thumbless grip will give you less control over the bar, but that will force you to have better bar balance and may keep you from spraining a thumb.

Keep your wrists rigid throughout the movement. Using wrist wraps [not straps] is a good idea.

To begin the movement, fill your belly with air, raise the bar off the pins and lock out your arms with the bar steady above your chest.

Pull your shoulders back and immediately lower the bar under control to your lower pecs just below your nipples. Keep your elbows slightly tucked on the way down. Do not drop the bar. The descent should take several seconds.

Never bounce the bar off your chest. Touch your chest with the bar and, after a moment, push it back up as you exhale. Keep your elbows tucked as you drive the bar off the bottom but allow them to flare out about halfway up. Keep your shoulders back and your chest spread throughout the movement.

Never lift your butt off the bench.

Never lower the bar to your throat or high on your chest.

Depending upon which feels best for you, the bar will rise vertically or at a slight diagonal (with two to four inches of horizontal movement) towards your head.

Unless it is your last rep or you are deliberately using a rest-pause technique, do not lock out your arms at the top. Go to just below lock-out and begin another rep.

If you fail to complete a rep, simply lower the bar to your chest, exhale, and slide out to the side.

The worst mistake with respect to doing a barbell bench press is to stop breathing, which can cause you to black out and drop the bar on your throat. Don't.

The second worst mistake is to fail on a barbell bench press rep outside a power rack and without spotters. If you ever have to roll a loaded barbell down your chest and stomach to get out from under it, you won't do that again.

What about auxiliary exercises to become better at bench pressing?

Probably the best are other kinds of bench presses (such as dumbbell bench presses), military presses, dips, chins (or pull-downs), and bent over dumbbell rows. Because strong triceps are a key to doing bench presses well, tricep pressdowns on a lat pull down machine should really help your bench press. Your pecs will power the bar off your chest and, as the bar rises, your triceps will do more of the work.

You may, if you want, use intensity techniques such as negative-only reps to become stronger on bench presses. To do them, lower a heavy bar slowly, have two spotters raise the bar for you, and then lower it again. If you do that once every month or two, you'll become stronger on bench presses. However, you never need to use negative-only reps and doing so is likely to increase the DOMS you experience.

Also, with all exercises except squats and deadlifts, you may train to failure at least occasionally.

It's likely that one side of your body is stronger than the other. Dumbbells are the best way to correct such strength imbalances. For that reason, doing bench presses and other upper body exercises with dumbbells for at least a couple of months is an excellent idea. Train so that the weaker side becomes stronger until it equals the strength of the formerly stronger side.

Assuming that you have access to sufficiently heavy dumbbells, the only problem you may have is getting into position. Either have two spotters put them into your hands after you are already on the bench or get into position as follows. Sit on the end of the bench with a dumbbell in each hand resting on one end just above your knees. Rock your torso slightly forward and then lie back onto the bench. As you do that, raise your legs to assist your arms in getting the dumbbells into the proper position. At the end of the set, just lower your hands and dump the dumbbells onto the floor.

First year trainees should never use fewer than 5 reps or 40 seconds on any exercise. Still, if you keep doing bench presses properly, it won't be long before you will be able to bench press your own body weight and that's a significant milestone.

The incline press may be considered a variation of the bench press. Like the bench press, it is done lying on a bench and may be done using either a barbell or dumbbells.

For safety, always do barbell incline presses in a power rack unless you have a spotter on either side. You may start the exercise at the bottom position by raising the barbell off the properly positioned safety bars.

Use a bench incline of either about 30 degrees or 45 degrees. If you have a short adjustable bench that also has a seat that adjusts up to prevent your butt from slipping off, you should use it set at the higher position. If you don't have such a bench, please don't set the bench at higher than 30 degrees.

The directions for doing barbell incline presses are similar to those for doing flat barbell bench presses. For example, at the bottom, your forearms should be vertical when looked at from both the front and the side. Don't lock out at the top of a rep and don't bounce the bar off your chest. When you press the bar up, its path will be similar to that of the path used during a flat bench press except that there will be less horizontal movement. Never exaggerate the arch in your lower back or use your legs for assistance.

Keep your feel flat on the floor while keeping your heels in front of an imaginary vertical line dropped down from your knees. It's important to ensure that your feet don't slip.

The dumbbell incline bench press has an important advantage over the barbell incline bench press because it allows your wrists to be in whatever is the most comfortable position for you. To get into position without spotters, use a technique similar to the one for getting into position for doing bench presses with dumbbells.

The first time you ever do them, incline presses will feel odd. However, after just a couple of workouts, you may well find that you enjoy them even more than flat bench presses and that they are more beneficial. (Personally, I think that flat bench presses are overrated and prefer doing inclines.)

52

9. Seated presses

The seated barbell press is an excellent upper body exercise that, when done correctly, is even safer than a standing or military press. It's the safest overhead press and it will really work your upper body.

The purpose of weight lifting is to increase your strength and quantity of lean muscle. That won't happen if you injure yourself. So please always ensure that you are using perfect exercise technique and the proper equipment so that your training will be safe as well as beneficial.

This exercise requires access to a sturdy, stable bench that can be adjusted to about 75 or 80 degrees. Do <u>not</u> use a vertical (90 degree) bench. Do <u>not</u> use a bench that is so high that it doesn't allow your head to go back slightly, especially at the top of the movement. (You won't have to think about this during the movement; your head will just naturally go back slightly.)

Some benches have an adjustable seat whose front can be raised to help prevent you from slipping down and off when pressing. If yours has such a seat, use it.

Put the bench inside a power rack. Center it so that you don't hit the rack's uprights while moving the bar. The barbell should be on pins set at the height at which you begin the ascent at the start of the exercise. Set the safety bars using the next lower pair of holes.

Commercial gyms sometimes have special pieces of equipment specifically designed for the seated barbell press. If your gym has one, it may work well for you, but it's more likely that it won't. If you don't have access to a suitable bench and a power rack, squat stands or spotters can work well.

Do <u>not</u> use a Smith machine for the seated barbell press. Its strictly vertical motion is unnatural and can cause shoulder problems.

Do <u>not</u> do behind-the-neck presses (or pull-downs on a lat machine). It's true that some trainees can do them for years without problems, but why risk it? Doing them can cause neck or rotator cuff problems as well as shoulder problems. The damage may not show up for many years and, once it does, it may be irreversible.

Keep your eyes forward during the movement.

Throughout the range of motion when doing a seated barbell press, keep a normal hollow in your lower back. This is the normal weight-bearing position for your backbone. If you exaggerate it, you are inviting injury. Simply keep your chest up and maintain a normal arch with your lower back.

When you're ready for your first seated barbell press, your feet should be flat on the floor and slightly wider than shoulder width. As with a bench press, keep your heels either directly beneath an imaginary vertical line dropped from the middle of your knees or slightly in front of that line. (If you pull them towards your head, you'll exaggerate the arch in your back.)

Do _not_ start a seated barbell press from too low a position or you will unnecessarily stress your shoulder joints. If you have shorter arms, you may start the movement at about the same height as your clavicles; if you have longer arms, you may start the movement at about the same height as your chin.

How wide a grip should you take? Have someone else ensure that your forearms are vertical when viewed both from the side and your feet at the bottom of the movement. In other words, at the bottom of a seated barbell press your elbows should be directly under your wrists. This is likely to be just wider than shoulder width. Once you find the proper grip position for you, use it consistently.

Use whichever grip you prefer. As with the bench press, you will probably want to wrap your thumbs under and around the bar. On the other hand, while a thumbless grip will give you less control over the bar, it will also force you to have better bar balance and may prevent you from spraining a thumb.

Do, though, use a pronated grip, which is one with your palms facing forward.

When you are ready, fill your belly with air and press the bar up vertically. Keep it close to your face without hitting your face. It's fine to lift your chin slightly as you begin to press upward. Come close to your chin without touching it with the bar. Do _not_ let the bar track forward.

Press evenly with your arms and shoulders. Keep the bar parallel to the floor at all times. Do _not_ let one hand get ahead of the other. This is especially important near the end of a set. <u>Especially when you get tired on any set, force yourself to focus hard to prevent technique deterioration.</u>

When the bar gets above your head, allow it to track slightly to the rear for a more natural movement. The horizontal distance will be about two or three inches.

Instead of resting by locking out your elbows, go to just short of lock-out and pause momentarily before descending. Inhale either during that pause or while descending, whichever you prefer.

Lower the bar under control; do not let it drop down. Do <u>not</u> lower it farther than your safe point or bounce at the bottom. Pause momentarily at the bottom before beginning the next rep and exhale during the ascent.

As with the bench press, keep your wrists rigid throughout the seated barbell press. Using wrist wraps [not wrist straps] is a good idea.

Keep your body tight throughout the movement. This especially applies to your legs, abs, buttocks, and back. Do <u>not</u> relax until the set is over.

What about auxiliary exercises?

Probably the best are the seated dumbbell press, bench press, incline press, dips, chins, back raises, core (midsection) work, and tricep work (such as pushdowns using a lat machine).

The seated barbell press is an extremely productive exercise. If you train intensely and regularly using perfect exercise technique, you are likely to be delighted with the results.

It's unlikely that you'll be able to do many chins (pullups) initially. Therefore, start by doing pulldowns on a lat machine. Once you are using 5% or 10% more than your bodyweight doing pulldowns, switch permanently to doing chins. So let's consider pulldowns and then chins.

Pulldowns are done in a lat pulldown machine. Normally, it will have a seat with an adjustable height and a padded, adjustable bar that goes across your thighs to hold you down. Adjust them to fit you.

There are different bar and grip options. Experiment to find which is most comfortable for you. Start with a straight bar, hands shoulder-width apart and supinated (palms facing you). Adjust the spacing so that it's not uncomfortable for your wrists and elbows. Also test a parallel grip with hands also shoulder-width apart (see the cover photo). Bars with knurling are easier to grip, especially when your hands get sweaty. By all means use some chalk on your hands.

Avoid using a very wide grip and avoid pulling down behind your head.

The exercise is simple. When you are properly seated, reach up and grip the bar. Keeping your eyes straight ahead or looking up, pull the bar down smoothly until it is the height of your upper chest and your hands are below your clavicles and raise it again. As you pull down, lean slightly back, but keep your back in the strength position, slightly arched, without rounding it; also, pull your shoulder blades down.

When your arms are nearly strait, don't rest: start pulling the bar down again. When your arms are extended, keep your shoulders tight and don't relax to get more stretch. Remember to focus on keeping in the sweet spot of the rep.

You may inhale when your arms are extended, hold your breath as you pull down, and exhale as your arms extend again. Alternatively, exhale as you pull the bar down. Towards the end of a set, take some extra, quick breaths.

As soon as your work set weight is slightly higher than your body weight, switch to chins.

Chins require an overhead bar. Ideally, it should be tall enough so that you are able to grip it while standing on your tiptoes. If it's not, you'll have to bend your knees during the exercise and, if you do, keep them at a fixed angle (so that they are not assisting you during the movement).

Initially use a supinated grip with hands about shoulder width apart. Experiment with a pronated grip with hand placement two or three inches wider than your shoulders. Adjust your hand placement so that it works well for you.

Do not use a wide grip and do not pull to behind your head.

Hang from the bar with your arms *almost* straight. Pull yourself up until the bar touches your clavicles or slightly lower on your chest and lower yourself down. Never drop back down or relax and stretch at the bottom. Keep the tension on. As in the pulldown, fully contact your lats by pulling your shoulder blades down. At the top of the motion, your back should be arched.

Inhale as you lower yourself and hold your breath when ascending and exhale at the top. Alternatively, inhale as your descend and exhale as you ascend.

As you get stronger, add weight. Never, however, add weight by hanging it around your hips. Instead, find a way to hang it around your neck. When you are only adding a little weight, using a rope may be fine. Later, you may need a chain wrapped with a towel.

Pulldowns and chins are extremely productive exercises. Why not master them?

11. Conclusion

This book contains all the information required for safe, effective, and efficient weightlifting for aging well physically from now until your dotage.

Unless used, understanding is useless. Mere theorizing is endless. Unless you are already following a good weight lifting program for aging well physically, if all you do is read this book and improve your understanding, you'll have wasted your time. The goal isn't to understand how to age well physically: it's to age well physically!

I've offered here both the general principles and the concrete specifics. What happens next is solely up to you.

If you are not already doing so, please get your physician's approval and get moving some poundages. You'll be delighted with your results.

If you want to train more than just one or two 10-minute workouts weekly or try a different routine, advanced beginner and intermediate programs are easy to find. Start with McRobert's book.

Thank you for purchasing and reading this book.

I've a favor to ask of you: please go to amazon.com, find this book's listing, and leave a review of it that will help others and may help me. Let others benefit from your judgment.

May you train well and be in good health!

About the Author

I was born 3 July 1946 in Teaneck, New Jersey, U.S.A. I graduated with a diploma from Blair Academy in 1964. I was a pre-professional philosophy major at Syracuse University and graduated in 1968. After two years as an Army lieutenant with overseas duty in Korea from 1968-1971, I attended graduate school at The University of Iowa where I received an M.A. (1975) and a Ph.D. (1977). Panayot Butchvarov was my dissertation director.

I taught humanities and philosophy at SUNY Geneseo from 1977 to 2009. I've authored over thirty books and been an Amazon Bestselling Author. I'm a former member of MENSA and the American Philosophical Association.

I played (full contact) hockey for many years in the Rochester Metro Hockey League; in my 30s I was a team Captain for two years and Alternate Captain for two years.

I meditate daily and joined Rochester Zen Center in 1994. I'm a certified life coach and also a certified energy healer.

My strength training partner and I are still going strong 1X weekly after about 30 years of training together.

Bass, Clarence. *CHALLENGE YOURSELF.*
Bass, Clarence. *LEAN FOR LIFE.*
Benson, Jon, and Venuto, Tom. *FIT OVER 40.*
Coleman, Ronnie. *HARDCORE.*
Darden, Ellington. *LIVING LONGER STRONGER.*
Evans, William, and Rosenberg, Irwin H. *BIOMARKERS.*
Haney, Lee. *LEE HANEY'S ULTIMATE BODYBUILDING.*
Holman, Steve. *HOME GYM HANDBOOK.*
King, Ian, and Schuler, Lou. *THE BOOK OF MUSCLE.*
Kubik, Brooks D. *DINOSAUR TRAINING.*
Lauren, Mark, with Clark, Joshua. *YOU ARE YOUR OWN GYM.*
McRobert, Stuart. *BUILD MUSCLE LOSE FAT LOOK GREAT.*
McRobert, Stuart. *THE INSIDER'S TELL-ALL HANDBOOK ON WEIGHT-TRAINING TECHNIQUE.*
Pepe, Larry. *THE PRECONTEST BIBLE.*
Reeves, Steve. *BUILDING THE CLASSIC PHYSIQUE THE NATURAL WAY.*
Schwarzenegger, Arnold, and Hall, Douglas Kent. *ARNOLD.*
Simmons, Louie. *THE WESTSIDE BARBELL BOOK OF METHODS.*
Strossen, Randall J. *SUPER SQUATS.*
Tesch, Per A. *TARGET BODYBUILDING.*
Venuto, Tom. *THE HOLY GRAIL.*
Wendler, Jim. *5/3/1.*
Yates, Dorian, and Wolff, Bob. *BLOOD AND GUTS.*
Zane, Frank. *FABULOUSLY FIT FOREVER EXPANDED.*

Not only am I a long-time strength trainee, but I'm also an experienced teacher.

Would you like a one-on-one, 45-minute telephone consultation with me? If so, I'll discount it to just $99. There are no guarantees, but none of my coaching clients has ever been dissatisfied. For more information, remind me of the deep discount and email me at dennis@endfearfast.com/

You might also have a look at my coaching website at: https://dennisebradford.com/

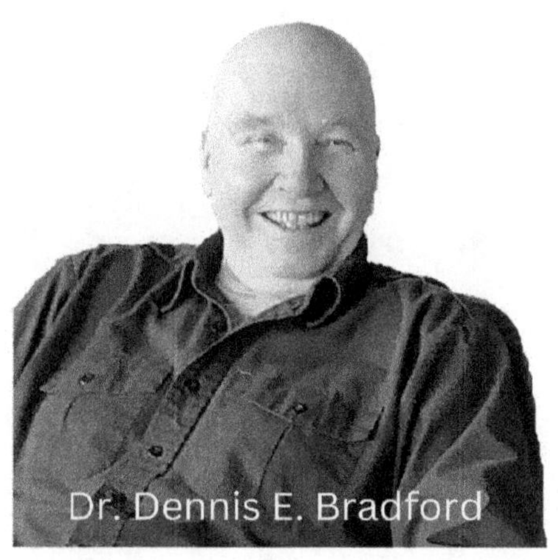